Health and Holistic Healing

Starting Your Own Wellness Store

Table of Contents

Chapter 1. Introduction

Step into the serene world of health and holistic healing as we embark on a fascinating journey of starting your very own wellness store! Welcome to our Special Report on Health and Holistic Healing: Starting Your Own Wellness Store. This immersive guide brims with cheerful optimism and motivating tales, mapping a step-by-step pathway towards launching and managing a successful wellness store. From understanding the nitty-gritty of sourcing high-quality, ethically-made products, to decoding the secrets of creating an inviting ecofriendly store ambiance - we'll unravel it all. With our Special Report as your guide, you'll not only join the burgeoning holistic health industry, but empower individuals to lead healthier, happier lives. Don't miss the opportunity to create a thriving business imbued with positivity, healing, and wellness. Light up your entrepreneurial spirit, and let's venture together into this prosperous journey of holistic wellness!

Chapter 2. Understanding Health and Holistic Healing

At the root of every successful wellness store, lies a solid comprehension of health and holistic healing. The interplay of these concepts sets the foundation for product selection, store atmosphere, and customer service.

2.1. The Basics of Health

Health, as defined by the World Health Organization, is a state of complete physical, mental, and social well-being and not merely the absence of disease or infirmity. Understanding this definition is critical to the operations of a wellness store.

Physical well-being relates to the functionality and innate vitality of the human body. This depends on factors such as balanced nutrition, regular exercise, sufficient rest, and preventive healthcare.

Mental well-being pertains to cognitive function and emotional resilience. It includes how we think, feel, and behave. Regular practice of mindfulness, learning new skills, creating and maintaining loving relationships and maintaining positive mental health are commonly recognized aspects.

Social well-being refers to one's ability to interact positively within social constructs and networks. Social connections, community involvement, relationships and good communication skills are important facets of social health.

2.2. Understanding Holistic Healing

Holistic healing operates on the principle that an individual's overall well-being is a direct reflection of their physical, mental, and emotional health. Rather than focusing solely on symptomatic treatment, holistic healing addresses the root cause.

Holistic healing encompasses various modalities. These may include natural therapies (such as homeopathy, naturopathy, and herbal medicine), modalities promoting physical wellness (like yoga, acupuncture, reflexology, and chiropractic care), and mental and emotional well-being approaches (such as meditation, mindfulness, and stress management techniques).

2.3. Your Store: A Facilitator of Health and Wellness

Your wellness store isn't merely a place that sells health products. Rather, it is a facilitator of health and wellness in all of its dimensions.

While it hosts a selection of goods designed to boost health and facilitate recovery, it should also aspire to be a tranquil haven that encourages individuals to invest time in their own well-being. Your store might offer comprehensive information about each product, workshops on health and wellness topics, or even spaces for holistic treatments and therapies.

2.4. Stocking High-Quality Products

Quality should be the guiding principle when it comes to stocking your store. Ethically sourced, natural, organic, and cruelty-free products make for trustworthy choices. Whether it's nutritional supplements, natural skincare, herbal teas, or therapeutic essential oils, each item should adhere to high standards of purity and efficacy.

By selecting such products, you promote not just the health of your customers, but also the welfare of our planet. Remember, part of health and wellness is respect for all living beings and our shared environment.

2.5. The Role of Education

Education plays a vital role in health and holistic healing. As a wellness store operator, part of your responsibility is to educate customers about different aspects of health, wellness, and the products you offer.

This can be done through informative leaflets, workshops, blogs on your store's website, or simple one-on-one conversations with customers. Making research accessible and understandable enables customers to make informed choices about their health and fosters a loyal customer base that trusts your store.

To sum up, understanding health and holistic healing is about recognizing the interconnectedness of physical, mental, and social well-being, and facilitating it through high-quality, ethical products, and education. This will help your wellness store to stand out as a beacon of health and healing in your community.

Chapter 3. Navigating the Market: Trends and Opportunities in Wellness

In the sprawling world of health and wellness, there's an undeniable vitality that not only nods at the sector's continuous growth but also the shifting consumer interests leaning towards holistic well-being. Advancements in digital technology, as well as our evolving understanding of overall well-being, pave the way for numerous opportunities within wellness, awaiting their turn to be seized by discerning entrepreneurs.

3.1. Analyzing Current Wellness Trends

Presently, the wellness industry is an amalgamation of varied facets - spanning fitness, nutrition, mental health, and personal care. The most notable trend in recent years has been the integration of technology within the wellness realm - inducing convenience and enhanced personalization.

Wearable fitness trackers, smartwatches, sleep monitors, and digital fitness platforms have substantially reshaped fitness, allowing an unprecedented level of customization. With real-time personal data at their disposal, users can tailor their workouts, measure their progress, and receive personalized health advice, which was previously not as accessible.

The surge in holistic approaches to health and wellness is another trend to keep an eye on. With roots in ancient cultures, holistic healing focuses on nurturing the mind, body, and spirit as interconnected entities. This shift from symptom-based care to proactive, preventative, and holistic self-care is seeing individuals consume more organic food, practice yoga, engage in meditation, and even explore alternative therapies like acupuncture or aromatherapy, leading to a dramatic demand increase for these products and services.

3.2. Opportunities Awaiting Entrepreneurs

With our understanding of the aforementioned trends, let's dive into the opportunities available for a wellness store in the current market scenario.

Consumers' rising interest in sustainable and ethically made products underscores an opportunity for wellness stores to cater to eco-conscious customers. Sourcing products that are not only beneficial for consumers but also for the environment can give your wellness store a distinctive edge.

Digital wellness is another opportunity ripe for exploration. Whether the product is wearable tech or an online platform that offers wellness programs and health coaching, ventures that consolidate technology and wellness are seeing a surge in popularity.

Lastly, the rise of holistic wellness indicates an opportunity to offer products and services across various wellness areas, ranging from organic foods and dietary supplements to mindfulness training resources and eco-friendly personal care products. Importantly, as consumers increasingly seek a one-stop-shop experience, a wellness store catering to all these needs stands in good stead.

3.3. Identifying Your Niche

Identifying and focusing on a specific niche in the wellness industry can lead to the creation of a truly unique business. This niche could be anything from organic skincare to posture-correcting fitness equipment.

In identifying your niche, it's worthwhile to conduct comprehensive market research, including comparative analysis of potential competitors, identifying gaps in the market, understanding consumer preferences and trends, as well as foreseeing potential market shifts. This can provide a clear understanding of the niche that represents the most profitability and sustainability for your business.

3.4. Building a Wise Business Strategy

Building a business strategy starts with a well-articulated business plan outlining your business's direction. At its core, it should pivot on unique value propositions that make your wellness store stand out amidst the competition and resonate with your target consumers.

In formulating your strategy, consider aspects beyond product selection. Think about your store's physical layout and ambiance, marketing and promotion strategies, customer service, and after-sales support. Adopting a holistic business approach resonates well with the essence of wellness.

Besides, it's paramount to integrate elements of sustainability and ethical considerations into your business strategy. Given the increasing consumer attention towards 'green' businesses that advocate for social and environmental causes, a sustainability-focused approach will add value to your wellness store and contribute to its long-term success.

The wellness industry is replete with multi-faceted opportunities. Leveraging the right trends, identifying a suitable niche, and building a robust, holistic, and sustainable business strategy can lay the foundation for a profitable and impactful wellness store. Our health and well-being are precious, so being part of an industry that nurtures them is sure to furnish not only economic benefits but the satisfaction of enabling healthier lives. What awaits is a journey laden with personal growth, entrepreneurial achievements, and the chance to contribute purposefully to the world of wellness.

Chapter 4. The Business Plan: Laying a Solid Foundation

Creating a robust business plan is the cornerstone of any successful business venture, and opening a wellness store is no exception. It's a comprehensive playbook that outlines your business objectives, market analysis, marketing strategies, and financial plans. It provides an efficient roadmap to help you navigate through your entrepreneurial journey.

4.1. Understanding Your Vision

First and foremost, clearly articulate the vision for your wellness store. This includes broad details about what you envision your business to be in the next five to ten years. Would your store be a local favorite or do you see it morphing into a chain of wellness stores across the state? Perhaps you aspire to take it online? Chalk out your dreams candidly for it keeps the entrepreneurial spirit alive and acts as a guiding star.

4.2. Defining Your Mission

Unlike the vision, the mission focuses on the purpose of your wellness store today. Your mission statement should reflect the impact you aim to have on your customers and community. Remember, your venture not just helps people buy wellness products but empowers them to lead healthier, happier lives.

4.3. Analyzing Your Market

A critical facet of the business plan is the market analysis. This reveals the potential of your wellness store in the current market. It entails exploring your target demographic, understanding their needs, and how your store can meet these needs. Investigate local competition and determine strategies on how to differentiate your store. It's also beneficial to keep an eye on wellness trends, both at a local and global level.

4.4. Setting the Right Goals

Goal setting helps to drive business growth and productivity. Set both short term and long term goals—each carrying its own significance. Ensure these goals are SMART: Specific, Measurable, Achievable, Relevant, and Time-bound. Regular tracking and evaluation of these goals should also be part of your plan.

4.5. Crafting Marketing and Sales Strategy

Stitching a powerful marketing and sales strategy is an absolute must. Your marketing plan should detail how your wellness store would attract and retain customers. It could include strategies spanning from social media advertising, SEO, blogging to hosting workshops and wellness events. On the other hand, your sales strategy should outline how your wellness store will convert prospects into customers and ways to upsell and cross-sell your products.

4.6. Detailing Operational Plan

An operational plan is a detailed layout of the day-to-day running of your wellness store. It includes sourcing of products, inventory management, store layout, and staff management. Sustainability being at the core of your wellness store, detailing how your operations will be eco-friendly will set you apart.

4.7. Deciphering Financial Projections

Finally, your business plan should comprise a sound financial forecast. Revenue projections, break-even analysis, cash flow statement, balance sheet, and profit & loss accounts are among the parameters to cover. It's crucial to remember that these estimates should be realistic and flexible to adjust with changing circumstances.

Building a successful wellness store might seem like a daunting venture, but laying a solid foundation via a comprehensive business plan can ease the process considerably. So wear your thinking cap on, put your best foot forward, and take the wellness industry by storm. Remember, this is not just a business, but a journey of healing, positivity, and prosperity.

Chapter 5. Sourcing Products: The Ethics of Holistic Health Merchandise

As the backbone of any successful wellness store lies an impeccable collection of products that not only promise beneficial health outcomes, but also resonate with the ethical values of holistic health and wellness. It's this distinctive product range that will be the core differentiator to your wellness store, establishing its character and building credibility amongst health-conscious consumers.

5.1. Ethical Sourcing 101

We live in a world that is hyper-aware of fair trade practices, sustainable sourcing, and ethical manufacturing processes. When choosing the merchandise that you'll be offering in your wellness store, it's essential that these factors take center stage. By ensuring your products are ethically sourced, you are staying true to the principles of holistic health - caring not just for the individual, but for the community and the environment as well.

To lay the foundations for an ethically sound inventory, learn to ask the right questions. Where does the product come from? Were any harmful chemicals used in its production? Were the workers involved in its manufacture treated fairly and safely? The answers to these inquiries will give you an insight into the true character of the products on your shelves and will guide you in your future business decisions.

5.2. Fair Trade Practices

Fair trade is dedicated to creating equitable international trading partnerships, based on dialogue, transparency, and respect. This means that the workers who create the produce and products you sell are paid a fair wage and work in safe and humane conditions.

Fair trade certification by organizations such as Fairtrade International or the World Fair Trade Organization can be a powerful signifier of ethically-made products, offering added assurance to your customers that their purchases reflect their own values.

5.3. Organic and Sustainable Products

In the world of health and wellness, organic and sustainably sourced products have always been of high value. Organic products are grown without the use of synthetic pesticides, genetically modified organisms, and irradiation. Meanwhile, sustainably sourced products take into account the long-term environmental impact of production.

Becoming knowledgeable about the certifications in your country will assist in identifying these products. Certifications such as the USDA Organic seal in the US or Australia's Certified Organic symbol are reliable indicators of organic goods.

5.4. Products with No Animal Testing

Another significant aspect of ethical sourcing involves ensuring that the products you supply have not been tested on animals. Many consumers today are vocal about their desire to purchase products that align with their ethical values, including respecting animal rights. Make sure to communicate with your suppliers to understand their product testing processes.

Companies that are certified by Cruelty Free International, PETA, or similar organizations, are often a safe bet. These certifications can serve as visible indicators of your store's commitment to ethical sourcing.

5.5. Responsible Packaging

Consider the packaging of the products as well. Packaging can be an enormous contributor to environmental waste, with single-use plastic being particularly harmful. Look for products that use minimal, recycled, or recyclable packaging.

Moreover, sustainability shouldn't stop at the products and their packaging. The store itself can be designed in an eco-friendly way using recycled materials, clever energy-saving features, and more.

5.6. Building Relationships with Ethical Suppliers

Your credibility as an ethical wellness store relies heavily on the relationships you maintain with your suppliers. Inquire about their sourcing methods, the principles guiding their business operations and ensure it aligns with the ethical values you want your store to uphold.

Establishing these relationships also takes a significant amount of research. Look for suppliers who are not merely motivated by profit, but who demonstrate a genuine commitment to ethical and sustainable business practices.

5.7. The Power of Local Sourcing

An often-overlooked avenue for sourcing ethical products is to look within your local community. Local artisans, farmers, and inventors sometimes produce high-quality, often hand-made goods.

By sourcing locally, you not just support local economy but also reduce the carbon footprint tied to goods transportation. Such partnerships also tend to be more transparent, giving you a clearer idea about how the products were made, who made them, and under what conditions.

5.8. Educating the Customer

Lastly, transparent and open communication with your customers is key. Embrace the responsibility of informing and educating your customers about your sourcing efforts and the product attributes.

In conclusion, curating an ethically sourced product range might be an uphill task initially, but the long-term benefits are worth it. Your wellness store will not just be a shop, but also a beacon of ethical, healthy, and holistic living. This will help you build a loyal customer base and position your store as a lead player in the holistic health industry.

Chapter 6. The Brick and Mortar: Designing an Inviting Store Ambiance

Creating an enticing store ambiance is not just about eye-catching interiors or dreamy color palettes; it's a comprehensive approach where every element plays its part in speaking your brand's philosophy. This holistic vision shapes the customer's journey, from the moment they spot your store till they happily walk out with wellness purchases.

6.1. Understanding Your Brand

The first and foremost step towards designing a store ambiance is understanding your brand. What is it that you're offering to your customers? What is your philosophy? Your design and aesthetic must resonate with your brand's ethos and the products you are offering.

A wellness store represents a calm, tranquil, and healthy environment. Hence, your store design should reflect the same. Nature-based colors, eco-friendly interiors, lighting to set a warm and inviting atmosphere can start forming a base of your store design.

6.2. Choosing the Right Location

Choosing a suitable location for your store is a substantial step. It must be in a place where your target audience often visits and is easy to reach. An easily accessible location not only brings in more customers but also helps in creating a better store ambiance.

Your store's environment is also significantly affected by the surrounding areas. A calming neighborhood, a serene park nearby, or even a busy shopping district can perfectly harmonize with your wellness store ambiance.

6.3. Store Layout

Chalk out a thoughtful store layout. Your wellness products should be organized and easy to find. Product placements play a vital role here. Popular wellness products can be placed at the front of the store, where they catch the customers' attention.

Similarly, related products can be arranged together. For instance, essential oils, scented candles, and aroma diffusers can be placed together to create a 'scent' section in the store. Walking through your store should be a journey of discovery for customers, where they can explore different aspects of wellness.

6.4. Aesthetics and Atmosphere

The aesthetic appeal of your store plays a significant role in drawing customers. Create an atmosphere that immediately hits the senses. Use a pleasing palette of colors that resound with tranquility and positivity.

Natural elements like indoor plants, water fountains, and sunlit spaces not only add a refreshing look to your store but also have a calming effect on the mind. Use of sustainable and recycled materials in your interiors will reinforce your commitment to wellness and environment.

6.5. Lighting

Well-thought-out lighting can make a difference in the overall look and feel of your store. Soft, warm lighting fosters a intimate and snug environment. Remember, the goal is to make your customers feel at ease and encourage them to explore and spend more time in the store. Strategically placed lights can be used to highlight specific product sections.

6.6. Aromas

The sense of smell is very closely tied to emotion and memory. Have a signature scent in your store that makes your customers feel welcome. It could be a calming lavender aroma from your essential oils section, or a refreshing lemongrass scent. However, ensure it is not overpowering, but subtly permeates the air.

6.7. Music

A shop plays a subconscious role in customers' experience. Choose soft, soothing music that complements your wellness store's atmosphere. Not too loud to overwhelm, nor too quiet to go unnoticed, it must strike the right chord with the ambiance.

6.8. Staff and Customer Service

Your staff plays a critical role in enhancing your store ambiance. Their warm smiles, politeness and readiness to help can set an inviting atmosphere. Regular training sessions will ensure they are well-versed in all the wellness products on offer.

Customer service goes beyond just providing information. Include spaces in your store layout where customers could relax, enjoy a detox drink or sample a wellness product.

6.9. Involving Customers

Make your store a wellness experience for your customers by

organizing workshops or live demonstrations. These could be yoga sessions, skincare or dietary advice from experts, or DIY home remedy workshops. These activities not only foster customer engagement but also deepen their understanding and commitment to a holistic lifestyle.

Without a doubt, every step in creating a wellness store ambiance requires a meticulous approach. However, the joy of providing a soothing environment for your customers, where they discover and embrace health and well-being, is truly rewarding. Your store will not be a mere retail outlet but a wellness hub, sprinkling good health and happiness in people's lives.

Chapter 7. Cultivating Connections with Suppliers & Practitioners

The cultivation of effective relationships with suppliers and practitioners is a key component of your wellness store's success. These relationships not only enhance your understanding of the industry but also provide access to a variety of high-quality products and services essential for your store. In this detailed guide, we'll traverse the lanes of communication, negotiation, understanding, and mutual benefit as we dive into the requirements of nurturing these crucial networks.

7.1. Identifying Potential Suppliers

The first step towards cultivating a rich network is identifying potential suppliers that fit your store's ethos and meet your product requirements. You need to consider various factors, such as whether a supplier adheres to ethical manufacturing processes, if they have a positive reputation in the industry, as well as their compatibility with your budget.

Industry events and exhibitions are excellent places to start. These events gather a congregation of potential suppliers, providing an opportunity to interact, network, and get a feel for their products. Additionally, online marketplaces, industry directories, and referrals from other retailers or individuals within your network can serve as valuable resources when searching for potential suppliers.

7.2. Building Trust with Suppliers

Once you've identified potential suppliers, you need to forge and strengthen relationships with them. This process begins with openness about your business intentions and future plans. It's essential that you appear inviting and empathetic while adopting a straightforward business attitude.

Ensure transparent communication about your terms, expectations, payment schedules, and any other contractual elements. Be punctual with your commitments, and responsive to your supplier's queries. Such behaviors not only cultivate trust but also lay the foundation for working out more favorable terms in the future.

7.3. Aligning with their Values

In the holistic health and wellness industry, mission alignment is crucial. When you align your business with suppliers who share your values around health, sustainability, and ethics, you can build stronger, more meaningful relationships.

To achieve this, identify the supplier's mission and values by discussing it with them or researching their website and promotional materials. If your missions are aligned, emphasize this common ground in your dealings to foster a shared approach to business.

7.4. Understanding the Practitioners' Needs

A crucial aspect of running a wellness store is the involvement of wellness practitioners. These might include yoga teachers, naturopaths, acupuncturists, or massage therapists, among others. Understanding their needs and ensuring that your store can cater to them effectively would lead to mutually beneficial partnerships.

Practitioners often require a platform to showcase their services and reach a broader audience. If you can provide this – perhaps with dedicated space in your store for workshops or treatment rooms for consultations – you'll be better equipped to attract and maintain partnerships with practitioners.

7.5. Fostering Partnerships with Practitioners

Forming partnerships with practitioners is more than just providing a space; it's about building a community. Events such as workshops, seminars, and health awareness initiatives not only attract customers but also provide practitioners an opportunity to interact directly with potential clients.

Creating such a symbiotic environment would differentiate your store, making it a hub for holistic health services. Remember, as your store becomes more popular among practitioners, it'll also become more desirable to customers seeking holistic wellness solutions.

7.6. Nurtifying Long-term Relationships

Your relationship with suppliers and practitioners should be seen as long-term partnerships rather than short-term transactions. Hence, always keep an open line of communication with them.

Regularly review partnership effectiveness, discuss any issues, areas of growth, and potential for greater collaboration. Appreciate their efforts and contributions to your store. These measures go a long way in nurturing relationships and retaining partners.

7.7. Negotiating Terms and Contracts

Irrespective of the strength of relationships, it's vital to frame clear terms and contracts. Be clear about price points, payment terms, delivery times, return policies for suppliers, and understand any regulatory compliances they must meet.

Likewise, with practitioners, establish clear guidelines about space rentals, schedules, and financial terms. Ensure all parties agree on the terms, significantly reducing the scope for future misunderstandings.

In conclusion, maintaining good relationships with suppliers and practitioners is a dynamic process – one that requires ongoing effort, transparency, and genuine interest in mutual success. By adhering to these guidelines, you'll create a thriving ecosystem for your wellness store, empowering individuals across the community – both suppliers, practitioners, and customers to lead healthier, happier lives.

Chapter 8. Marketing Your Store: Digital Strategies for the Wellness Niche

In the competitive world of wellness retail, visibility is key. The landscape of marketing has evolved with the advent of digital mediums, making it crucial for your business to adopt strategic online practices. In this exploration, we will traverse ways to position your wellness store in the digital space, delving deep into targeting, content strategies, social media, SEO, email marketing, and more.

8.1. Understanding Your Target Demographics

Before launching any marketing efforts, you need to understand who your target customers are, their attitudes, behaviors, and how they engage with digital media. Utilize data analytics tools like Google Analytics and Facebook Insights to gauge the demographic and psychographic information, creating your ideal customer persona. Having a clear picture of your potential customers will guide you in crafting your digital marketing strategies effectively.

8.2. Digital Content Strategy

Content is king in the digital space, and its curation should reflect your brand identity, ethos, and the value you wish to provide your customers. Blog posts, guides, how-to videos, podcasts about health, wellness, and holistic healing not only position you as an industry expert but also help in boosting your SEO efforts.

Ensure your content is relevant, engaging, and caters to the needs and interests of your target audience. Pay attention to trends and advances in the wellness sphere and map your content accordingly. User-generated content or UGC is another powerful tool; it creates a sense of community and boosts credibility.

8.3. Leveraging Social Media

Social media platforms like Instagram, Facebook, and Youtube are potent tools for wellness companies. They not only act as channels of communication but also offer unique ways to showcase your products. Use Instagram to share beautiful visual content - from product features to behind-the-scenes glimpses into your operations or sourcing process.

Facebook is ideal for distributing content, engaging with customers, and running targeted advertisements. YouTube offers an excellent platform for long-form content like interviews, guides, or tutorial videos. Regular content updates, quick responses to comments, and user engagement are essentials in maintaining an active and vibrant community.

8.4. Search Engine Optimization (SEO)

SEO is all about improving your website's visibility to those searching for the products or services your store offers. Focus on optimizing your website content and structure with relevant keywords, meta descriptions, and alt-tags. Also, consider the user experience on your website; factors like page loading speed, mobile optimization, and ease of navigation can impact your ranking on search engine results. Regular, high-quality content like blog posts or wellness tips can also enhance your SEO efforts.

8.5. Email Marketing

Despite the multitude of digital channels available, email remains an efficient, direct, and personal way to communicate with your customers. Collect email IDs through website pop-ups, checkout steps, or specific lead magnets like free e-books or guides. Send out newsletters or updates on new products, wellness tips, and personalized recommendations, ensuring content is personalized and not overly salesy. Also, consider automated email responses for cart abandonment, re-engagement strategies, or post-purchase follow-ups.

8.6. Paid Advertising and Influencer Collaborations

While organic efforts are vital, paid advertising can give your online visibility a robust thrust. Platforms like Google AdWords and Facebook Ads allow highly-targeted pay-per-click (PPC) campaigns to reach your desired audience. Influencer collaborations are another way to create trust and gain access to an already engaged audience. Choose influencers whose values align with your brand; the collaboration will appear more genuine and resonate better with followers.

Marketing in the digital domain is a mix of using the right channels and strategies to reach your intended audience. Consistently learn, adapt, and maintain an open dialogue with your customers will keep your wellness store at the forefront of their minds. Harness the power and reach of digital strategies, and watch your wellness store flourish in the marketplace.

Chapter 9. Building a Community around Your Store

Building a community around your wellness store is an integral aspect of your business's success. It goes beyond transactions to build relationships, foster trust, and create a loyal customer base that resonates with your values and trusts your brand. Here's a detailed guide on how to go about it.

9.1. Defining Your Mission and Vision

Before you start to build your community, it's essential to clearly define your mission and vision. What values does your wellness store embody? How do you plan to impact the world positively through your store? Answering these questions will provide a roadmap and help you share a consistent message that attracts like-minded individuals.

Your mission statement should succinctly explain what your store offers, who it's for, and how it differs from competitors. Meanwhile, your vision statement should communicate your long-term goals and the impact you want to have on your community. Once clearly defined, ensure these messages permeate every aspect of your business, from product development to customer service.

9.2. Cultivating a Unique Store Identity

With your mission and vision in mind, you can now proceed to craft a unique brand identity. This identity sets you apart in the market and strongly resonates with your target group. To create one, consider factors like your store's aesthetics, your products, your communication tone, and your staff's attitude. An important aspect of this is to create a welcoming and positive atmosphere as this strongly aligns with the wellness industry.

9.3. Building Online Presence

In today's digital age, building an online community is just as important, if not more, than building a physical one. Start by building a user-friendly website complete with an e-commerce platform. This allows customers who can't physically visit the store to purchase your products.

Social media platforms serve as invaluable tools for community-building. Start by creating profiles on popular platforms such as Facebook, Instagram, Twitter, and LinkedIn. Use these platforms to share helpful content, announce new products, or promote upcoming events. Also, interact with your audience by responding to comments, reposting their content (with permission), and thanking them for their support.

Engage with influencers in the wellness industry to boost your brand's visibility. This can be through collaborations on blog posts, social media takeovers, or jointly hosted events.

Email marketing is another effective platform to interact with your community. Regular newsletters sharing wellness tips, product information, or store updates can keep your brand at the forefront of customers' minds.

9.4. Organizing Community Events

Community events serve as a way to bring customers together, allowing them to connect over shared interests. This could range from wellness workshops and seminars to fitness classes and health fairs.

These gatherings should deliver value to participants and provide opportunities for them to interact with your products. Successful events can lead to increased customer loyalty, brand visibility, and ultimately, sales. Also, consider charity events that align with your brand and can contribute positively to the community.

9.5. Networking within the Industry

Staying connected with other businesses in your industry can present several opportunities. Attend trade shows, wellness expos, and local business events. These networks can lead to potential collaborations, partnerships, or co-hosted events.

9.6. Customer Service and Engagement

Exceptional customer service can't be overlooked when building a community around your wellness store. Ensure all customer interactions, whether in-person or online, are pleasant, helpful, and in line with your brand.

Engage with customers beyond transactions. Show genuine interest in their wellness journey, ask for their feedback, and take their suggestions seriously. Remember, your customers are at the heart of your community; keeping them happy and engaged is key.

9.7. Building a Loyalty Program

Lastly, a customer loyalty program can help keep your customers coming back. Happy customers are likely to become advocates for your store within their own social circles, indirectly expanding your community. Provide occasional discounts, birthday benefits, or points that can be accumulated and redeemed.

In conclusion, building a community around your wellness store means getting involved with your customer's welfare on a personal level. It means giving them a platform to voice their opinions and ensuring they feel part of your brand. With a clearly defined mission, a unique brand identity, and a dedication to engaging your customers, you're well on your way to creating a tight-knit community around your store.

Chapter 10. Ensuring Success: Customer Service and Satisfaction in the Wellness Industry

The journey of successful entrepreneurship in the wellness sector requires more than just dreams or even high-quality products. It thrives on the cornerstone of exceptional customer service and satisfaction. You, along with your entire team, need to understand that every single customer is unique, and their needs and expectations are diverse. Ensuring customer satisfaction in the wellness industry involves recognition and respect of that individuality and establishing firm, trust-based relationships with your valuable customers.

10.1. The Power of Empathy

A term often thrown around in the customer service industry is empathy. To empathize essentially means to step into another's shoes, to understand and share their feelings for that moment. In the wellness industry, empathy takes on a critical role. Your customers may approach you with an array of wellness-related concerns, pain, and worried questions. Train your staff to assist every customer with genuine empathy. This means understanding the customer's problems, anxieties, and offering service and products that truly address their personal wellness needs. Natural empathic responses can help you build a loyal and satisfied customer base.

10.2. Building a Capable Team

Empathy is a quality to be valued, but it's not enough on its own.

Your wellness store team must have comprehensive knowledge and understanding of the products and services you offer. Build a capable team who can help your customers make educated choices. This includes mastering the art of attentive listening and honing the skill of effective communication to adequately address customer queries and concerns. Regular training sessions, workshops, and staying up-to-date with the latest industry trends will be essential to ensuring superior customer service and satisfaction.

10.3. Introducing Personalized Experience

Personalization is a proven strategy for improving customer satisfaction. When customers feel special and well-understood, they are more likely to frequent your establishment and recommend you to others. Implement customer data management systems to store customers' purchase histories, preferences, and personal details such as birthdays, anniversaries, etc. Utilize this data to offer tailored recommendations, deals, and personalized greetings during their special days. It's these little gestures that build up a customer's affinity towards a wellness store.

10.4. Ensuring Product Quality

A customer's trust in your wellness store is direct feedback for the quality of products and services you provide. Adhere strictly to essential quality standards – ensure that all products are safe, ethically sourced, and provide the promised wellness benefits. Be transparent with your sourcing and quality control methodologies to win everlasting customer trust.

10.5. Prioritizing Post-Sale Service

Once a purchase is completed, don't let close contact with your customers dwindle. Post-sale services such as timely delivery, customer-friendly return policies, and post-purchase follow-ups to ensure they're satisfied with the product can make a difference. Ensure seamless communication channels for customers to voice their concerns and feedback. Immediate resolution to their problems fosters trust and leaves a lasting impression.

10.6. Implementing Omnichannel Approach

In today's era of digital connectivity, an omnichannel approach towards customer service can instill instant gratification and satisfaction. Make your wellness store's products and services accessible across various touchpoints - brick-and-mortar, website, social media platforms, and even home delivery. A seamless, integrated experience across these platforms enhances user convenience, and gradually, customer satisfaction.

10.7. Listening to Customer Feedback

Whether positive or negative, every piece of feedback is valuable. Maintain diverse avenues for customers to provide feedback – suggestion boxes at your physical store, interactive website forms, regular customer satisfaction surveys, and more. Assure your customers that their voices are heard and meaningful changes are implemented based on their feedback. This transparency will help you instill trust and cause an uptick in the satisfaction levels of your customers.

10.8. Nurturing Customer Relationships

Consider fostering relationships and creating a sense of community among your customers. Organize wellness workshops, product launches, and special wellness events that encourage your customers to interact, learn, and grow together. The sense of belonging nurtures stronger relationships between your wellness store and your customers.

Seamlessly combining the touch of empathy with personalized service, post-sale assurance, an omnichannel approach, and nurturing relationships, while welcoming feedback forms the foundation of successful customer service strategy in the wellness industry. Remember, a satisfied customer is not just a testament to your customer service success but also a brand ambassador propagating the value and quality you represent. It's no longer about how many customers you serve - the focus should be on how well you serve. And that's the secret formula to creating a thriving wellness business driven by customer satisfaction.

Chapter 11. Paving the Future: Sustainable Practices for Wellness Stores

In the ever-evolving retail landscape, sustainability has emerged as a significant facet, influencing both business practices and consumer choices. As we embark on the journey of establishing a successful wellness store, the incorporation of sustainable practices becomes paramount. This commitment to ecological integrity while managing a thriving business speaks volumes about your dedication to the holistic wellness ethos.

11.1. Sustainable Procurement

Arguably, the most influential aspect of sustainability in retail is procurement. The choices you make in sourcing products can have a far-reaching impact not only on the environment but also on the consumers you serve and the ultimate success of the store.

When sourcing products, consider the provenance of the items you stock. Choose to collaborate with suppliers who are transparent about their materials, processes, and principles. Look for seals of approval such as Fair Trade, Organic, or Rainforest Alliance, which can give you and your customers assurance about the ethical and sustainable nature of the products.

Consider the packaging, too. Are products excessively packaged, or do they utilize eco-friendly materials? Plastic-free and zero waste options are increasingly popular with health and wellness consumers. Make a conscious decision to provide alternatives that contribute positively to the environment.

Select items that are made from recycled, upcycled, or renewable sources, given the choice. Every little bit counts in this quest for sustainability, and a product's lifecycle can be an important part of your store's narrative.

11.2. The Store Layout and Design

Next, consider your store's physical premises, the layout, and how it is designed. Lead by example and show that you are practicing what you preach.

Optimize your store layout for energy efficiency. Open-plan designs can help in natural lighting, while insulation can help control temperature, which can, in turn, help reduce energy consumption.

Recycling is not just for products; it can be implemented in the shop fit-out, too. Utilise reclaimed materials for fittings or countertop surfaces, and consider sourcing second-hand furniture as an environmentally friendly practice.

Consider the lighting in your store. Opt for energy-saving bulbs or LEDs. These not only consume less electricity, but they also last longer, reducing the frequency of replacement.

11.3. Green Energy

Transitioning to green energy is another step to a more sustainable practice. Green energy systems such as solar panels may significantly minimize your business's reliance on fossil fuels. Moreover, it also sends a strong message to your customers about your commitment towards ecological preservation.

Your investment in sustainable energy systems could also draw in customers who are eco-conscious. Furthermore, it could reduce energy bill costs in the long run, making it a worthwhile investment.

11.4. Waste Management

Efficient waste management is a cornerstone of sustainable practice. A conscientious commitment to reducing, reusing, and recycling can greatly reduce the environmental impact your store has.

Create a comprehensive recycling system within your store. This includes having designated bins for different materials such as cardboard, plastic, and organic waste.

Assess your store's waste production regularly and identify ways to reduce it. For instance, partnering with suppliers who have returnable packaging schemes can drastically decrease the amount of waste generated.

11.5. Employee Practices

Sustainable practices aren't just about products and policies; they are also about people. Employees are your best ambassadors; hence their understanding of and commitment to sustainability is vital.

Host regular training sessions to ensure your team understands what sustainability means and why it's important. Encourage them to practice sustainability both in-store and within their own lives.

Allow employees to give their input on sustainable practices. Creating a culture of sharing might make your store a pioneer in implementing new ideas that even bigger brands haven't considered yet.

11.6. The Power of Community

Engage with the local community and inspire them to tread on the path of sustainability. Collaborate with local schools and organizations to host workshops and events focused on sustainable living. Inviting guest speakers to discuss topics such as climate change, renewable energy, and waste management can help educate and inspire your customers.

11.7. Communicating Your Commitments

Transparent communication about your sustainability efforts is key to building trust with your customers. Make information about your suppliers, energy use, waste management, and community engagement readily available. This could be in-store, on product labels, or through your website and social media channels.

It's equally important to encourage feedback. Let your customers know that you want to hear their ideas and respond to their concerns. This will not only help you improve, but it also involves your shoppers in your sustainability journey, creating a sense of shared responsibility and community.

By implementing these sustainable practices, you pave the way for a successful brand that's defined not only by profit margins but also by its environmental and social consciousness. Your future wellness store will not just be a beacon of health for individuals, but for the community, and our planet itself. As we remember, wellness is not just a state of body, but of our environment too. Sustainability is not an option anymore; it's the only way forward.

www.ingramcontent.com/pod-product-compliance
Lightning Source LLC
Chambersburg PA
CBHW071044260726
48661CB00007B/3154